THE SEA FOR SPIRITUAL MEANING AFTER BRAIN INJURY

This is book 2, and is often referred to as the "Light" book.

It is a sequel to "*A View from the inside, A survivor's perspective*", which is called the "dark" book. The first book is an insightful, raw look into what happens to many brain injury, stroke and concussion survivors during the first couple years.

A series of essays

Contents

Building a New Me

After writing about my experiences of pain, depression and the constant war within between the old me and the new, I took a couple years off to ponder the changes that I had between the old and new me.

It was now a full 7 years after my brain injury and stroke and I had fully come to terms with the grieving over the old me and all the losses that I had experienced on two levels, more on that later.

This book, and much of my findings, are more than just personal experiences. Over the past several years, as facilitator in two brain injury support groups, and being active in several social media brain injury and stroke support groups, I have been listening, journaling, comparing, and remarking over the many similar experiences and emotions that survivors share.

There were the physical aspects such as the constant vertigo, pain, brain shocks (or lightning strikes), and medications that help with the pain, but add to the dizziness. Constant vertigo makes it nearly impossible to walk without a cane, and tactile pain over one side of my body make it hard to touch, grasp or be touched.

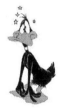

There are social aspects, old friends who knew the *old me* were largely unable to handle the "death" of the *old me*, and I could see that my loss was too great for them to work out in their own minds. I am one of the lucky few who have found so many new friends who did not know me at all before my brain injury. Still, when I try to regale them with stories of my high-achieving pre-injury life, I can see the disbelief in their heart.

I can't drive or work anymore, but somehow this does not seem to matter to my **New Me** friends.

The **Old Me** had cultivated many relationships where individuals could depend on me: to be someone who cared, to be someone who helped, and in the last 5 years of the **Old Me**, to be their pastor.

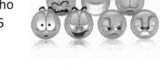

The **New Me** has found friends that I must depend on. People who will care for me, people who will help me, and people who will listen to me.

My last several years has been a journey of building a **New Me** that still works hard to be all that I can be in each moment, but allows for help from others to bridge the moments.

Building a **new me** requires drawing up plans and blueprints for activities that I have never tried and many that I have never enjoyed before, and allowing myself to scrap and start over as often as it takes until I discover the right set of **New Me** experiences that matches my new physical, emotional and spiritual self.

PLEASE, NO PLATITUDES, NO CLICHES,
...My filters are turned off.

Before continuing into the important subjects, I need to clear the air about two things that I find personally upsetting, and want to assure you that my approach in this book will have neither.

I want to comment about "Filters" and platitudes and clichés. One way of defining Filters is to say that it is the way that we make sure that we don't say the wrong thing at the wrong time.
But we also use "Filters" to accept other people's opinions, even when it upsets us. We use filters to keep from reacting when we think that someone is responding with useless or unhelpful words, and instead, just nod with respectful smiles.

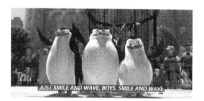

After surviving a brain injury, concussion or stroke, a person's filters are damaged. Sometimes the failing filters will increase as other symptoms improve.

When filters are damaged we will often speak the "truth" that is in our mind without being filtered by such things as caring about the feelings of others, or being concerned about our surroundings or situations. We can unintentionally initiate strong words to ask a question or for help, or act out in either personal or group settings with unusually forceful or mean statements. What comes out is often the difference of what a non-brain injured person often thinks, and is willing to say. God help us if everyone could read each other's minds!

As I continue in this book, I will demonstrate that, like some many other aspects of surviving and growing, handling filters is a spiritual art, not a physical or mental exercise.

Platitudes that don't speak to our reality such as "You look like you are walking really good lately" (I'm walking with a cane), or "You're talking just fine" (when it took me 5 minutes to convey 1 sentence), can go from hurtful to insulting.

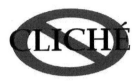

Cliches, well meaning words that everyone hears others say that is supposed to be meaningful but are quite painful.

So, NO, everything DOES NOT work out for my or your <u>COMFORT</u> .

No, Time will not heal everything, there are no brain transplants.

No, I am OVER IT yet, and I probably will never be, but I am fighting every day to get THROUGH IT.

THE CENTRAL QUESTIONS AFTER SURVIVAL:
Who am I to be for now on?
and
What will I do for now on?

AFTER THE GRIEVING IS DONE.

A Cutting.

It is the blade below the thorn,
On which the rose's sorrow is borne,
Ne'er to return healing power to the nest,
Separated before its time to thus bless,
The plant which begets its love thorny,
Continues, knowing only grief and glory.

T. Schuck

After my incident, which involved both a brain injury (VAD – vertebral arterial dissection) and ischemic stroke), I found strong validity in the concept that my life would be divided into almost two distinct lifetimes.
There was the "**old me**", all the life, dreams, plans, and abilities that existed before my incident, and now the "**new me**", which is in many ways, is still in the process of discovery. After all, it has only been a few years in development.

There was a hard, and very difficult grieving process. Part of me had died, and died hard. There were the immediate and obvious losses to grieve, the loss of balance, visual normalcy, driving, work, normal walking, freedom from pain, independence, etc.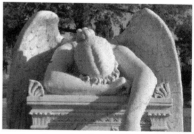

But then there were the latent losses. After my dysphonic voice began healing and I started to talk in a normal voice, I found that my well trained, experienced, tenor singing voice was gone. Prognosis: gone forever.

I discovered that even though I have reasonably "dealt with" the grieving process that is largely inevitable in such life altering changes, that there would be some deep lasting emotion, that because we must live with our own memories, can never be completely hushed.

STILL SORROWS RUN DEEP

There is a sorrow that permeates the core of the survivor. I suppose I cannot single out the brain injury and stroke survivor as having deep sorrows, and I wonder if it is present in all those whose loss is without ending.

This sorrow is as far removed from depression as the notion of true joy is from temporal happiness. Depression affects the immediate mood, numbs the character to reality and pushes the body and mind into conclusions and actions that often just increase the depression, or seek to harm the person.

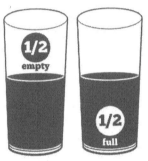

Take a large drinking glass and fill it ½full with water. Take a glass that is less than a ¼ the size of the first glass and have a large bowl ready to pour into. Now look at the large glass. Is it half full or half empty? Many will argue that you can find out if you are a pessimist or optimist by your answer. But I say, neither, you are using the wrong glass. Now take the large glass, hold it over the small glass and over the bowl. Pour the large glass into the small glass. It will overflow into the bowl.

Look at the small glass. It is full. It is all that you can hold, it is completely you, all that you can be and do. But what about everything that was dumped out, everything that was suddenly lost? Those I call the "Deep Sorrows".

Deep sorrows are the remnants of who we were before some cataclysmic event occurred in our life. For some, it is the pain and loss of a loved one, a spouse, parent or child in a horrific manner. Or the loss of everything we held dear in a violent storm. But the deepest sorrows are often reserved for the loss of self, loss of limbs, brain injury, stroke and the like. It is the ocean of all we were meant to be suddenly cut off without warning. Sometimes it is the memory itself of who we were. The disconnect of the person you are today to the person that made you who you are.

It is the sorrow of poets and of the painters. It is one of the many doorways that I will discover opening to me that causes me to take a spiritual journey after my stroke and brain injury.

Our sorrow stems from a loss of ourselves, a death of who we were. Even if we did not make retirement plans, or plans for 10 or 20 years from now, all of our plans probably envisioned abilities and capabilities that were much more than this.

And now with much of life spent living day to day with pain and neurological issues, it is painfully difficult to look at any future at ask "is there more?". Any desire to answer "yes", has to involve our spiritual side, which must be stronger than our body and mind in order to answer "There is more!"

YOU CELEBRATE WHAT???

Look again at the small glass**. It is full. You are a complete person. Filled to the brim. Overflowing. It can be the new you.**

Many survivors that I know, including myself, actually celebrate their survival date (when they woke up in the hospital) in preference over their birthdate. This includes all the elements of a birthday celebration such as cake, friends and decorations. All of this is designed to help the survivor and their community realize how important the "new me" person of the survivor is and will become.

But some survivors go beyond that. Since some friends, relatives and survivors themselves cannot release their relationship to the "old me" memories of the survivor, the survivor now finds themselves in a constantly awkward state of relationships.

Family and friends either can't or won't let go of their own memories of the person that they knew, and they fight bitterly to keep their memories of the "old me" alive even though the survivor is now incapable.

The result is that in extreme cases, healing was found by the family and friends, and the survivor, holding a type of funeral ceremony for all the memories of how the survivor used to be. Where every person could eulogize their love and loss of the person that they knew, and hopefully make commitments to the new person, the survivor, standing there. Even the survivor will eulogize him or herself, talking of the dreams and desires lost and then with flowers and beautiful customs, the "old me" would be laid to rest.

A wake would follow, with the survivor as the guest of honor.

Again, none of this resolves the body, or the mind, but it opens another door to take on the spiritual journey after stroke or brain injury.

Psychologically, I prefer simplicity, and of all definitions of "what makes us human", I prefer the simple viewpoint that each of us is made up of:

The Body: The Physical
The Mind: Intelligence. The Thinking, critical, logical, reasoning
The Soul: Feelings, love, hate, our connection to Eternity

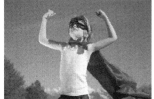

Before my brain injury and stroke, I would often place much higher significance on the first two, in varying degrees. As a young man, I loved the outdoors, scuba diving, hill climbing, horses, and trails. I also loved to workout at the gym. I was gifted with natural intelligence, I never had to really "work hard" at school, yet maintained a 4.0 average.

As I grew older, I discovered that my intelligence, thinking and problem solving skills could earn me a lot a money, and my life and retirement looked great and secure. Boil it all down, I was all about success.

My soul was doing pretty good. I have always been a family man with old style 1950's family values. I have always been a spiritual man, faithful to my beliefs and working hard to honor God in myself and others.

I don't really remember ever thinking hard on this question, but I am certain that I now know the answer:

Required to make a choice, which would it be:
- keep the Body, but lose the Mind and Soul;
- keep the Mind, but lose the Body and Soul;
- Keep the Soul, but lose the Body and Mind?

But then of course, the brain injury struck.

And, in many ways, it feels like both the question was posed to me, and the choice was made for me.

The first obvious impact was the body. I felt devastated in that area. The first morning in the hospital, not knowing what happened and no one around, I tried to get out of bed, only to discover that I had no strength in my left leg, collapsing to the floor.

Physical Therapy still continues as a constant reminder that my deficits will keep me from ever being who I was or wanted to be.

The second loss came as I struggled with concentration, mental focus, and memory loss. Mathematical algorithms that used to be "fun", were now impossible and painful to read. My ability to process data was damaged. I

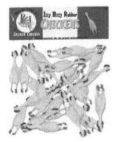

attempted to return to my original work, only to discover how much damage had really been caused, as brain shocks and seizures became the standard response to challenging situations. Although I cannot understand or decipher all of the technical data on a MRI report, I am certain that it must allude to the fact that my brain now looks like a bag of rubber chickens.

I am able to focus on my body by performing my physical therapy tasks, and I am able to focus on my brain by keeping it alert and challenged with writing, photography and jigsaw puzzles on my computer and tablet, but all of these exhaust me quickly, causing mental fatigue, common among many survivors

What I am most able to focus on, without any inhibitions, is my spiritual journey, asking questions of myself, of what some call "Providence", or "Higher Power" or "God" and listening to good audio books. Reading is difficult due to eye focus problems.

It may take months or years to repair the body and the mind, but I can repair and focus my spiritual journey much quicker. I can seek answers to important topics that my deep sorrow is focusing onto now – my value, the value of others, love, caring, beauty, good and evil, kind and harsh.

I admit, this is not something that is quick or easy to face – as is chronicled in my first book, my own journey from injury into the depths of loss and despair - but at some point, if we dare to hear it, we must face these three facts:

1. Our body, which feeds information to our mind and is designed to perform tasks when signaled by our mind, now has broken pathways, and is not reacting properly.

2. Our mind, with the excess overload of trying to compensate and find new pathways is hurting, constantly hurting.

3. If I am going to start over, to build a new me, I should start where I can show real progress.

There are two mottos that I have come by that I have made my own:

> Real People, Real Issues, NO PLATITUDES

I can't tolerate platitudes, or clichés, or cheezy sayings. Just because I walk slow, or talk slow, or react slow, does not mean that I think slow.

> There is More

There has to be more. More than just rolling over and playing dead. I will not accept defeat. I will not accept that I am a worthless leach on society, even though my contributions may be no greater than refrigerator art. But there is also more spiritually. There is something greater than all of this. Some purpose, some goal, some reason.

HARSH BEAUTY

Don't speak lightly to me of easy beauty,
Of simple cares, and perfect blessings,
Where every cloud is lined in silver
And everything works out for the best.
For I know.
I know of harsh beauty and volcanos,
Of thunderstorms and the lightning bolt
That sets a green forest ablaze.
And the coastal shore
Pounded by the hurricane waves.
I see a beauty that is both
Rich in the awesome and aweful.
For I know
I see the beauty in a damaged person
A wheel-chair, walker, or a cane,
A voice torn out of their brain,
Muscles that cannot hear the heart.
For I know
As you are now, we once were,
As you think now, so we think now.
Same speed, same way, same thoughts.
Its only disconnected at all the externals.
For I know
Physical Pain that shall not relent
For I know
We still see beauty
Maybe more intensely than you shall ever know
For I Know
Don't talk to me of casual beauty
That costs nothing and hurts little.

<u>For We know</u>

In the poem on the previous page, I attempted to capture both of the thoughts that I expressed previously: (*real people, real issues, no platitudes*) and (*There is more*).

In *Harsh Beauty*, I describe beauty through the eyes of pain. Beauty exists, but it is harsh, it is not always roses and sweet sunsets. You either accept it for what it is or you run from it.

We cannot run from it, because we live it.

Yes, *we know*. Because we are unable to turn our eyes from the man or woman in the wheel chair, or holding the cane (it is ourselves in the mirror), we are forced to look. We also look at others very differently too. We learn to empathize with pain. We know life exists joyfully (not always happily) in spite of pain, during pain, through pain, sometimes inspired by pain. There is still laughter, thoughts, desires, wants, needs, plans, hopes, EVERTHING. Our spirit is very much alive.

Origins of the Search for The Spiritual

I am going to digress back to *WHY*, the origins of the search of spirituality, and I hope this may even be interesting to those who have no interest in "religion" or "faith" as it is commonly used.

Perhaps one of the most striking, as in "hard hitting", aftershocks of survivorship is the sudden role reversals that take place. Some abrupt and some plodding, the survivor of severe neurological trauma discovers that while their physicians and physical therapists focus rebuilding their nervous systems, the survivor must make stock of who they are as a person even within their family.

For many the first role reversal comes in the form of independence and reliance. Survivors have often built a lifetime of careers, families and relationships ***developing themselves as someone that others could rely*** on for help, that others could depend on, that others could see as role models of independence and ethics.

The suddenness of a single event such as a brain injury or stroke reverses all that, sometimes with no warning, but seldom without a fight. If the physical prognosis requires the survivor to accept their new life, that "fight" period not to give up the old life is often marked by depression, mood swings, even thoughts of suicide.

The most difficult, yet most crucial life skill is holding onto or finding personal value in these role reversals. To be perfectly honest, many "rewarding tasks" that are offered to the survivor may feel like offering pony rides to a war horse.

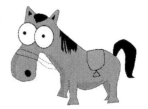

Finding a meaning and purposeful life inside of all role reversals is a life-changer, in as much as it requires you to make life changing choices.

The survivor has to actually set aside all their years and successes and make the choice that they are no longer an accountant, computer programmer, architect, construction engineer, or self employed business owner.

Maybe now they are a book reader, listener, life journalist, painter, observer of nature, conversationalist. Vocations that were surreal and unnatural to them before, now become a whole new life purpose.

I personally went through so many failed vocational ideas of what I might do in my "New Me". I purchased oil paints, I thought I might become a great oil painter. Didn't happen.

I bought books on origami. I thought I would become a learned person on origami and help others learn it and enjoy social interaction that way. Didn't work out.

I bought a camera. I wanted to take pictures of birds.
Birds move too fast. My eyes don't focus that quickly. So I decided maybe I will photograph every plant and tree and discover some unknown wildflower. In doing this project, I discovered the delightful squirrel.

Now, I take thousands of pictures of squirrels. I've published three fantasy books about squirrels.

All you need is Faith and Trust

And a little bit of pixie dust.....

Trust and Faith in others, which at one time in our lives were really just sweet platitudes, now take on personal significance, as the survivor *must* choose to trust others rather than their own brain and will, believing (finally) that their thinking processes are flawed and dangerous. Looking out for number 1 now means giving up your most prized possession, your "TRUST". It is the one thing that we learn in life that we are never to give away lightly.

Survivors from spiritual, faith, and ethical humanistic backgrounds ENJOYED the ability to DO something within their systems, either out of gratefulness for life, blessings, eternity, second chances, or dutifulness to secure a chance at eternity and second chances and receive blessings.

Certainly, one does not have to be a believer in any particular faith or religion to rush to the front lines of a terrorist, hurricane, tornado or earthquake disaster and start helping the victims and hurting immediately.

In all my wonderings and wanderings, what I have found is that

There comes a point in one's existence,
And especially for those survivors
who reach a determination
that there are too many questions,
too many problems,
all too great to give up trust to another human for answers,
that they need to find something or some ONE
that is higher, smarter, and more trustworthy than people.
This is what I call the beginning of the survivors search for
Spirituality.

To be sure, there are those who never have need for spiritual answers, I do not know why. I cannot give you a response why some have no search for spirituality, especially after a life altering event such as stroke or brain injury. I have no argument. I'm too stupid. I plead brain damage

More of the people that I have encountered who have been assaulted in mind and body such as me, find themselves on a spiritual journey. I like to think that is why you are reading this little book.

Do we Need God to Exist?

In my personal experience and from all that I have heard and read from others, it appears to me that brain injury, stroke and intense neurological pain demands several things of us.

It causes us to divide our life between our "old me" and our "new me" . This is not a cliché, and I apologize for repeating it so often, it is valuable truth.

It causes us to redefine, rebuild, or create belief systems that are much more real, personal, relevant, **and with zero nonsense and pretense.**

I don't have time or stamina for platitudes or for a stained-glass God.

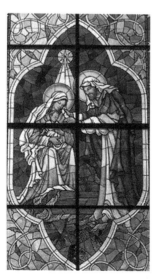

If God does exist, and in all my research, there is an overwhelming consensus that "HE MUST EXIST!", then my brain, our brains, now somewhat removed of social impediments, will now have a whole new set of constructs about our expectations and needs

First, no more distance. We were already too close to meeting God in person for there to be distance now. Spiritually, we know that The God that exists must be close, always ready to hear me,

Second, no more shame. Spiritually, our new me, understands, that the God who exists is real, bigger than my emotions, can take ALL of my questions, anger, pain, hurt, bad attitudes, love, hate, joy, sorrow, crying spells, EVERYTHING, and still want to be my GOD. God does not get emotional or check out because he cannot handle our rants or loss of filters.

Third, no more changes. Just because people change and leave, our new me perceives that the God who exists is permanent and unchanging. To us, sudden changes in personal relationships often create sensory overloads and are unbearable to our brain. Changes are frustrating, get me anxious and give me headaches. The God who exists is one who can be Trusted.

Fourth, no more platitudes. I probably already have every Chicken Soup book that even come close to my situation, and have heard every uplifting adage and bible passage that is known.
Spiritually, I know that the God who exists will send me friends that show how much they care, not how much they know.

I can accept that most of the time He might do these things through people that have walked close to Him for years, but I get nothing out of them just posting words on Facebook or reciting phrases out of context.

I'm not dumb, I Know God is not Santa Claus, and is not my personal genie, and I don't want a God who is. I want a God who runs the universe His way, and does not take my advice, NOR ANYONE else's.

Part II: What Should He Be Like?

While riding in the car with my wife the other day, she was trying to explain something that she had heard on the news to me, and I had to finally ask her to just STOP talking.

"If it doesn't directly impact our eternal destiny or squirrels, I just can't deal with it right now."

She reminded me that I neglected to include our marriage in that list. *Whoops, My bad*. I quickly corrected my statement.

In any case, my statement was that I get easily overwhelmed and befuddled, and I often remind myself that there are really very few things that matter.

Ok. Squirrels shouldn't matter that much, but I'll plead brain damage and let's move on.

As I wrote in my earlier comments, I was formulating that I wanted a relationship with God that was based on no-silliness assurances of eternity that did not require a perfect body and brain and that did not require me to perform like a circus ape or complete a number of tasks from a check off list from someone's interpretation of a passage or two of the Bible.

If God existed, and my body and mind were subject to major damage and were not the save havens that I thought they were, then I needed to start living and thinking God-centric, what was best for my spiritual health and rebuilding.

Not that I am willing to stop enjoying family, and vacations, and friends, and shopping and squirrels and flowers, and all the fun things that I do enjoy just yet.

I found a relationship with God that actually works, a very personal relationship. A healing one. But I'll get to that later.

Survivor Serenity Prayer

God, grant me the serenity
To accept the things I cannot change, Courage to change
the things I can, and wisdom to know the difference.

ACCEPTING THE THINGS THAT WE CANNOT CHANGE

And not becoming distressed or depressed over them, Such as:

1. Many survivors of brain injury or stroke survivors, or those with lifelong neurological disorders have to cancel or limit vacations, outings with the family or date nights with their spouses because of a sudden onset of symptoms. It is also common to have days of being restrained to bed due to pain.

2. You are not unique, and although it could not have come at a worse moment, you cannot change it. This is part of who you are, and although you cannot change this, there are other things that you CAN change. Please learn to accept this about yourself.

3. For many of us, the demands of our old career, possibly any normal career, are now beyond our capacities, both intellectually and functionally. .

4. Pain and other symptoms are what define your medical condition, that is a fact, they are NOT what defines the person that is YOU.

5. You may not have the PHYSICAL stamina that you had before, you may tire easily.

6. You may not have the INTELLECTUAL stamina that you had before, you may get headaches quickly.

7. You may not have the EMOTIONAL stamina that you had before, you may get overwhelmed quickly.

COURAGE TO CHANGE THE THINGS THAT I CAN CHANGE.

1. You can communicate what clues you will use to those who are closest to you when you are reaching the point of no return and need to leave or rest. My wife and I can be with a group a people laughing and enjoying ourselves, when suddenly, what seems like "out of the blue", I will turn to her and say "I'm done". This means that I URGENTLY need to get away and to find a place of rest immediately, and she needs to help get me there. I also have learned that it's OK to say that I just had an unexpected "attack", and we'll have to reschedule our dinner out. These things happen, and we adjust.

2. My old career involved software design and managing people, both of which are impossibilities for me now. Before my brain injury and stroke, I never thought I would enjoy photography and painting miniatures, but they have become my new hobbies and my new life. It took me a while, and courage to discover this new life, but its well worth it.

3. When my wife sees me obviously trying to control the pain, she will ask me "are you going to be all right?" my answer usually is "of course, are there any other options?"

4. I challenge myself to the end of MY physical stamina, not the end of a "normal" person's stamina, and you know, I still feel pretty good.

5. I make sure I avoid intellectual requirements that will cause headaches, like figuring out the tip on my bill at the restaurant, I ask someone else to do that for me. Or pretty much any math, I don't do math anymore, I let others do it for me, it causes a severe brain burn. But I really do enjoy art, history, and pretty much anything that is rightbrained. I guess that tells where the damage is and where it is not.

6. I use all sorts of communication clues. My favorite phone introduction is "I have a brain injury, but I need to discuss this, so let me ask this". I usually find this opening statement almost always disarms the other person.

AND THE WISDOM TO KNOW THE DIFFERENCE

1. It is not a wise decision to respond to your embarrassment over having to leave early or cancel appointments by isolating yourself from everyone for FEAR of having to leave again. You need to let people understand that this is who you are, and let them accept this about you. Don't isolate!

2. Don't get blinded by discouragement over loss of career that you refuse to find new hobbies or interests.

3. Find support groups, talk to others like yourself. Acceptance without Courage will lead to depression. Courage without acceptance can lead to harm later. Try to understand and know the difference.

4. Don't believe what your heart and mind tells you anymore. They are both so messed up. Constant chemical and electrical fluctuations are now mostly responsible for telling you lies about love, about what someone just said, or the way they said it, or what they meant when they said it. You have to work out a defined set of core values and beliefs and call that "truth". Then gauge every thought and emotion against that truth.

THE DECLARATION OF INDEPENDENCE.

I hold THESE truths to be self-evident

You have to form your own Declaration of Independence from the tyranny of your brain injury. You cannot allow your brain injury and a simple set of imbalanced chemicals and electrical impulses to manipulate your life and emotional health. That is why I recommend that you create a declaration of TRUTHS THAT ARE SELF-EVIDENT.

This is my declaration. Yours may have parts removed, added or changed. Everyone is different. As long as you really meditate hard on it.

1. I believe in God in heaven, and in His Son Jesus, that they have a plan for me.
2. I did not deserve what happened to me, this is NOT punishment, it is not to make an example of me
3. I do NOT blame God for my trauma, but I see that God is still able to love me and be active in my life regardless.
4. Accidents happens to everyone, one happened to me.
5. My Wife loves me
6. My Oldest Son loves me
7. My youngest Son loves me
8. I have real friends who care for me.
9. I have enjoyed many real fun experiences since my injury
10. I will continue to enjoy them as long as age and illness allows
11. A good attitude makes good friends, complaining drives them away.

My independence under attack

I have to admit. Every day, sometimes every moment, these 11 truths are challenged.

My brain will tell me:
- *Your wife is angry, she does not love you anymore. Run!*
- *God has abandoned you*
- *Your kids really don't care about you, they have their own lives*
- *You will never have another good day again.*

And many, many other lies.

If your truths are not absolutes, then you are sunk.

SURVIVOR PERSONAL RESPONSE CHART

It is my own personal chart, I don't think one chart fits all people, my chart might not be a perfect fit for you.

	Postive Attitude	Negative Attitude
Pain	Cry a Little	Cry a little longer
Loss of Memory	Live for Today	Can't remember the happy good old days
Headaches	Can't do nothing about it	Focus on it
Confusion	Enjoy my inner Squirrel	Work hard on trying to focus
Dizziness	Enjoy my inner Squirrel	get all bummed
Can't talk right	Enjoy my inner Squirrel	get all frustrated
Can't walk Straight	Enjoy my inner Squirrel	walk a lot less
Losing Balance	Enjoy my inner Squirrel	sit a lot more

Please Stop worrying

Oh, please stop asking me, are you OK. The other day, I was walking, with obvious ataxia and without my cane, around a place with friends, when I had a two left feet stumble. Someone said "Are you OK". I responded. "I'm ok, this is how I walk without my cane". Then they asked "Do you need your cane?". I politely replied "No", and then I slowly repeated "This IS how I - walk - without a cane". They understood, that I meant that I was getting along fine, I did not want the burden of the cane for that moment, but my choice came with the ataxia.

I think you know how this feels. You feel freedom from your devices that support you, but your friends and family want to protect you and see your departure from your devices as dangerous.

And when we see someone who does not act, or behave the way that we want them to, we want to have them caged or wonder who let them loose on us.

One huge change that has occurred in me since my brain injury/stroke is that I really don't pre-judge anyone without first knowing their entire backstory. Hence, my next poem:

The BackStory.

EVER NOTICE HOW EVERYBODY IS NOBODY
UNTIL YOU TAKE TIME TO LEARN THEIR
BACKSTORY?
I DON'T JUST MEAN THEIR STORY,
WHAT COLOR THEY LIKE, THEIR FAVORITE TEAM,
OR WHAT THEY ATE TODAY,
A SHARED RECIPE, PICTURES OF THE KIDS.
THAT STILL DOES NOT MAKE NOBODY
SOMEBODY TO YOU.

BUT THEIR BACKSTORY DOES,
WHAT THEY HAVE LEARNED IN LIFE.
THE PAIN THEY HAVE ENDURED AND OVERCOME.
THE PAIN THEY ARE ENDURING AND YET LAUGH
AS YOU DO.
WHAT THEY HAVE LOST.
WHO THEY HAVE LOST.

THE STRENGTH THAT COMES FROM HAVING NO
STRENGTH

YET PRETENDING TO HAVE ALL THE
STRENGTH IN THE WORLD
ALL THE TIME IN THE WORLD
THEIR BACKSTORY THAT MAKES THEM YOUR HEROES
THAT MAKES THEM SOMEBODY
TO THINK ABOUT, TO CARE ABOUT ,
TO REMEMBER,
AND TO PRAY ABOUT.

What does this poem say to you? How does it make you feel when you see others or when others see you and write you off as a disabled person not worthy of their time? Our united message is clear, through Facebook groups, community groups, and support groups, walk-a-thons and other events we try to educate the general public that we are worth their time, that we are gracious, loving caring people, with wonderful, beautiful backstories.

JOHN 16:33 AN APPLICATION FOR SURVIVORS

Why do bad things happen to good people is not a question for survivors, for "bad things" and "good things" have become truly relative. There is only What we were, Who we are, and today.

What we were is fading or lost to memory.
What were are is a path of discovery that is new, and started out very, very cruel; but hey, now we're coping
Today is what we have to write our journal in.

Fuhgeddaboutit? : The word is on the exit signs as you leave Brooklyn NY. What does it mean to me?

"Do not worry about it; it does not matter; it is beyond your control. Do not waste my time with such notions

Although some may misinterpret I AM better than that, there is a double meaning here. First, it is clearly ascribed to GOD, (Jesus), and second, the believer can assert that they can do all things through Christ who strengthens them.

In This world you shall have

Pain
Memory Loss
Disastors

FUHGEDDABOUDIT

I AM | Better Bigger | Than That!

God (Jn 16:33 Para.)

The Survivors Bill of Rights

It could be easy to mistake the Survivors Bill of Rights as a list of items that I believe that survivors have the right to impose on their loved ones, family, friends, caregivers, and society in general.

Nothing could be further from the truth of the origin of why it was developed.

Survivors, more than anyone, are given to appreciate their role as receivers, and although gratitude is truly at the heart of every survivor; pain, confusion, inability to express oneself clearly, etc., make it often seem that survivors are more about themselves and less about gratitude.

But survivors clearly understand what it is like to be on both sides. Before their own personal trauma, they used to observe other survivors and wondered about their motives for actions.

But I do digress.

The Survivor's Bill of Rights is written for the encouragement of Survivors. I simply wrote It to say, "You can stop feeling guilty" as guilt is a significant pattern in the life of a survivor.

It appears on the next page

THE STROKE / BRAIN INJURY SURVIVOR'S
BILL OF RIGHTS

WE BELIEVE that all survivors are now endowed with a certain inalienable rights by the fact that they have survived through the grace of God, strength of will, the support of someone, and the advances of medicine, a complete SNAFU in our brains.

1. To be incomprehensible in our speech, and hope you to be listening
2. To be scrambled in our thoughts and hope you to be understanding
3. To be defenseless against physical pain and hope you to be patient
4. To be powerless against emotional stability and hope you to be supportive.
5. To random hissy fits, tantrums, crying's, because we are defenseless in our pain OR powerless in our emotions
6. To chocolate at any time, dessert before dinner, and plenty of treats for all the reasons mentioned above
7. To be treated like a "normal" person when it suits us
8. To be treated like a "disabled" person when it suits us

9. To mourn our old life, old skills & old ways
10. To mourn the fact that we can't remember anything about our old life, skills or old ways, except they must have been better

Searching for Spiritual Meaning

The search for spiritual meaning, I believe, must have these three elements:

1. It is achievable. It can be stated as an objective and an achievement. My mind and body are slow to heal, but my spirit is something that I CAN work on

2. It involves making a personal decision where your spiritual journey will find its best outcome. Will it be in finding a relationship with a real God who is interested in relationships? Will it be a different journey?

3. It will contain for you, the place or person that you can confidently go, to find answers for the questions that have no answer

Simply put, in my declaration of independence from the tyranny of my body and mind, I have placed my faith in, and thereby created a core truth for myself: I am a follower of Jesus Christ. All that He said is true. Jesus is the Son of God, He is God the Son, His message to his followers is profound and sometimes difficult, but the eventuality is, as one writer put it "absent in the body, is present with the Lord".

What about Jesus and my four basis needs?

➤ Jesus said he will be with us forever, living with us, that we can call on him and he will answer

➤ Jesus accepted the one who denied him and the one who doubted him, he was fond of the hurting and the shamed

➤ It is said of Jesus that He is the same yesterday, today and Forever

➤ Jesus disliked hypocrites the most, and cared physically for needs

I hope your search for spirituality will be as successful as mine!!
If you want to know more, please email me at wincss@yahoo.com , or facebook me at tom.schuck.7

Made in the USA
Middletown, DE
22 January 2022

59431316R00022